VOCAL POWER

HOW TO DEVELOP YOUR VOICE

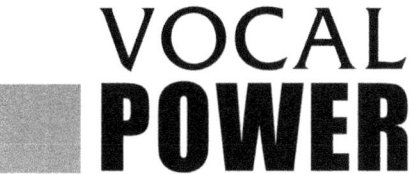

VOCAL POWER

HOW TO DEVELOP YOUR VOICE

revised edition

christina kaya

kayaco
seminars

VOCAL POWER
HOW TO DEVELOP YOUR VOICE, Revised Edition

Copyright © 2003, Kayaco Inc.

First edition printed 1989

First printing March 2003
Second printing November 2003
Third Printing September 2015

ISBN: 978-0-9219961-2-5
LSI Edition: 978-1-4600-0587-3
E-book ISBN: 978-1-4600-0588-0
(E-book available from the Kindle Store, KOBO and the iBooks Store)

National Library of Canada Cataloguing in Publication

Kaya, Christina,

Vocal power : how to develop your voice / written by Christina Kaya ;

illustrated by Magdalena Kaczynska. -- Rev. ed.

ISBN 0-921996-12-8

1. Voice culture--Exercises. I. Title.

PN4162.K39 2002   808.5   C2002-905541-5

Illustrated by Magdalena Kaczynska

To order additional copies visit:
www.essencebookstore.com

For seminars and online workshops visit:
www.KayacoSeminars.com

Printed by *Essence Publishing*. For more information, contact:
20 Hanna Court, Belleville, Ontario, Canada K8P 5J2.
Phone: 1-800-238-6376. Fax: (613) 962-3055.
E-mail: publishing@essencegroup.com
Internet: www.essencegroup.com

For Andreia and Rosalind

TABLE OF CONTENTS

*"Let thy speech be better
than silence or be silent."*

Dionysius the Elder

INTRODUCTION

When you hear an outstanding speaker, do they know something you don't? Dynamic speakers have almost certainly taken time to develop a most essential component of their communication system—their voice. Your voice is an integral part of your image and you are judged to a great extent by the way you speak. Your level of education, personality traits and social position are all determined not only by what you say, but how you say it. This may not be fair, but it is true.

In business, politics and other circles we have all seen good ideas fail because the speaker appeared to lack conviction and we have also seen bad ideas succeed because they were well presented. Of course, content is important, but so is the presentation! To date, there have been many psychological experiments that demonstrate that this is true. We are all influenced in our decisions by many things beyond just the information presented—including the quality of the vocal delivery.

This book presents a vocal development program that will help you develop the ability to express conviction, emotion, and subtlety of thought to connect in a meaningful way with other people. Being able to connect with people and influence them is a powerful capability, hence the title of this book, "Vocal Power."

Because your body is essentially your "instrument", the exercises involve making sound and moving your body. We all recognize the need for physical exercise to keep our bodies in shape. Similarly, it follows that vocal exercises will help you to develop and maintain an expressive, dynamic voice.

The vocal exercises in this book will help you improve the clarity, tone quality, and projection of your voice. It is important to note that this book is not intended to address major speech defects such as extreme hoarseness or any type of throat pain. A physician should be seen in person to examine anything that you reasonably think requires medical attention. This book is for people who have average, healthy voices but would like to develop their voices to be more expressive and dynamic for personal success in their chosen careers.

The exercises are presented in an order that is logical to the learning process, so it is best to learn and practice the exercises in the order in which they are presented. Always approach each exercise gently. Don't work on any one exercise too long. If, at any point, your throat feels rough, you are either overdoing the exercise or you may be doing it incorrectly. Read the instructions again. If you have a cold, or if you feel tired on a particular day, then skip practice for that day. Your body is not a machine and you must allow for fluctuations in energy and general physical condition.

Who can acquire a dynamic voice? Anyone can. Great voices do not usually happen by chance. Like most worthwhile achievements, a good speaking voice is achieved through patience and practice. You will not have to wait until you have completed the whole book to experience changes in your voice. Every exercise improves some aspect of the quality of your speech. Over time, the changes you experience in the exercises will form new habits and your voice will reach a new level of expression and power. I hope you enjoy working through this book. The results should give you a great deal of satisfaction, both personally and professionally.

YOUR VOICE

What kind of voice do you have? We all use our voices differently in different situations. The way we speak to a child sometimes differs from the way we would speak to a colleague, client, or employer. We can often tell from the "formality" of tone quality whether someone is speaking to a stranger or a friend. Many people have a "telephone voice". Do you?

It is a difficult task to evaluate our own voice objectively. We hear our voice differently from the way others hear it. You could gather opinions on how your voice comes across by asking friends or acquaintances, or you could get a more technical and accurate appraisal from a voice coach. However, the easiest way to get a personal "snapshot" of your voice is to listen to your voice mail or make a recording of your voice, including an announcement of the date, so that you can compare it with a future recording.

What are you listening for, and what are the characteristics of a good voice?

1. Easily heard and understood
2. Natural
3. Expressive
4. Dynamic

First of all, you should be easily heard and understood. Is your pronunciation clear? Do you speak too quickly or slur words together? Do you speak loud enough? Do listeners have to work to hear what you say? Or is your voice too loud? Very often our hearing regulates the volume of our voice. Whenever a client contacts me with reports that their voice seems to be too loud for people, I suggest they take a hearing test before spending money on voice classes.

Your voice should sound natural. If voice training results in your voice sounding affected, over-enunciated, or unnatural, we have defeated the purpose. People are wary of others who come across as though they are covering up something or trying to be something they are not. We all have an innate sense of what is "real".

A key objective of voice training is to develop expression that enhances the meaning of the content or information we are presenting. An expressive voice, capable of conveying conviction, passion, or subtle thought, holds attention and connects with people. The goal is not to develop "one voice", but a voice that is like an instrument—capable of expressing different feelings, depending on the context.

An outstanding speaker has a dynamic voice that projects a sense of their personality and feelings without sounding forced or uncomfortable. When we choose to speak to people it is for more than just information. If we decide to go beyond writing to communicate with others, it is often to motivate, persuade, or affect some kind of change. These goals are reflected in the meaning of the word "dynamic".

DYNAMIC:

1. Action
2. Bring about change

Many people ask how long it will take to change their voice. Some of the exercises, as many have experienced in my seminars, produce an immediate effect. Then, the effect "wears off" as the usual, familiar way of speaking takes over. People assimilate change at different rates and, with voice work, your body is learning as much as your mind. I have clients with clear goals and tons of will power who have made significant, permanent changes that are noticeable to others after just three months.

You may wish to record your voice so, in a few months, you can hear how it has changed. Start the tape by indicating the current date, then read a paragraph from a book, magazine, or newspaper, or just talk about something. Keep this recording and compare it to another recording three months from now.

"If I was given eight hours to chop down a tree, I would spend seven of those hours sharpening my axe."

Abraham Lincoln

THE SPEECH PROCESS

How does your voice work? Unlike most other physical processes, vocal production can't be "seen." You can't watch your diaphragm muscle "develop" or see your vocal cords "vibrate more efficiently." Voice clinics that treat specific vocal problems have equipment that can videotape your vocal cords as you speak and the "quality" of your voice can be represented graphically on a computer.

A detailed study of the anatomy and physiology of sound production isn't necessary, but some explanation of your sound making apparatus will help you understand the purpose of the exercises.

Every sound-making device requires:

1. Power or energy
2. Vibration
3. Resonance

For example, when playing a violin, plucking or bowing the string supplies power. The string vibrates and the body of the violin resonates to amplify the sound. The sound bounces around inside the hollow cavity of the body, amplifying the vibrations of the string. The sound exits through the holes in the body of the violin and you hear the sound.

A violin sounds much fuller and richer when played by a concertmaster than when played by a novice. It may be the same instrument, but the concertmaster has learned to play the instrument to maximize the quality of the sound produced. Similarly, you can learn to play your "vocal instrument" to maximize the quality of the sound.

In human speech, breath is the power or energy, vocal cords are the vibrators, and the cavities of the body are the amplifiers or resonators. Unlike musical instruments, people do not just make sound—we use language to express ourselves. So human speech has a fourth component—articulation. This is the manipulation of the mouth (lips, tongue, and palate) to shape sound into a meaningful form—words.

The co-ordination of your breath, vocal cords, throat, lips, and tongue produces your voice. The way you use the components of your vocal apparatus is established early in life and evolves partly by copying those around you. Dialects and accents are learned the same way—by copying the speech examples in the surrounding environment, which is why a Texan speaks differently than a Nova Scotian. The quality of your voice is also determined, to some extent, by your personality. A shy person does not usually have a loud voice.

People attach personality traits to different types of voices, and an underdeveloped voice, or a voice with certain faults may cause your personality or abilities to be misperceived. A monotonous voice does not necessarily mean a person is boring. A breathy voice may sound weak or indecisive, although to some it may sound sexy. A person who mumbles can leave the impression of being lazy and indecisive.

The first set of exercises will help you improve your articulation and also open up the point of release for your sound—your mouth.

ARTICULATION

Your listeners must be able to hear everything you say without strain. When addressing people at a distance, who can't see the movement of your mouth, articulation is even more important. People pay attention to a person with clear, articulate speech; an articulate speaker is perceived as being more decisive than someone who mumbles.

Clear speech depends on the efficient co-ordination of movement of the lips, tongue, palates (hard and soft), and teeth. Articulation exercises will remove tension, improve flexibility, and strengthen the "moveable" components in speech: the lips, tongue, and soft palate, so they are able to form words clearly, with a minimum amount of effort.

You can test these muscles with some tongue twisters! Many have tried tongue twisters for fun, but tongue twisters have been used for a long time to improve pronunciation skills. One of the most famous, "Peter Piper picked a peck of pickled peppers…" can be traced back to a 1674 publication in London, England, entitled: "Peter Piper's Principles of Plain and Perfect Pronunciation."

Tongue twisters use repetitions of sounds that employ certain muscle groups to determine which muscles may be weak and test our ability to switch quickly from one sound to another.

Read the following tongue twisters aloud and put a check beside the phrases you find difficult. You could also record yourself reading the list.

You will be aware of which tongue twisters trip you up or make you "tongue twisted" and you will also hear which consonants are not clear in your speech.

1. Strange statistics.

2. Quick coke kick.

3. Choose stew Tuesday. Tuesday is stew day.

4. For fine fresh fish phone Phil.

5. Miss Smith dismisseth us.

6. Is this a zither? This is a zither.

7. Betty beat a bit of butter to make a better batter.

8. I often sit and think
   And fish and sit and fish and think
   And sit and fish and think and wish
   That I could get a cool drink.

9. The dude designed the desperate plot to dupe the dreadful desperado.

10. When does the wristwatch strap shop shut?

11. Which wristwatch straps are Switz wristwatch straps?

12. Slim Sam shaved six slippery chins in sixty-six seconds.

13. She stood on the balcony inexplicably mimicking him and welcoming him in.

14. The sixth sick sheik's sixth sheep is sick.

15. How many cuckoos could a good cook cook if a good cook could cook cuckoos?

16. The horse's hard hoofs hit the hard high road.

17. It isn't the hunting on the hills that hurts the horse's hoofs. It's the hammer, hammer, hammer on the high road home.

18. Violet vainly viewed the vast vacant vista.

19. A tree toad loved a she-toad that lived up in a tree. She was a three-toed tree toad, but a two-toed tree toad was he.

20. Around the rugged rock the ragged rascal ran.

21. Willie's wooden whistle wouldn't whistle.

22. Whistle for the thistle sifter.

23. Black bug's blood.

24. Rubber baby buggy bumpers.

25. Nine naughty nanny goats nibbling nine nice new nasturtiums.

26. Three thick thistle sticks.

27. If a dog chews shoes, what shoes would he choose to chew?

28. Fresh fried flesh of foul.

29. The juggler juggled and jiggled juice in a jar.

30. Peter Piper picked a peck of pickled peppers.
    A peck of pickled peppers Peter Piper picked.
    If Peter Piper picked a peck of pickled peppers,
    Where's the peck of pickled peppers Peter Piper picked?

Difficulty with any of these tongue twisters may indicate certain consonants may not be as clear as they could in your daily speech. You may have also identified certain sound combinations that you find difficult. Read them again after you have completed the articulation exercises.

For your interest, articulation exercises also help achieve other accents or dialects. We all develop muscular habits as we grow. The ease with which we form certain sounds or our difficulty with others reflects these habits. Anyone who learns to speak another language experiences difficulty in forming sounds that do not exist in their "mother" tongue.

For example, many languages do not require the sound "th" and many students of English will substitute "d" or "z" instead, as they have difficulty co-ordinating their teeth and tongue to form "th". Certain accents will result in "take zem to ze uzzer side". Similarly, English-speaking students have the same trouble when trying to speak another language, which requires sounds that do not exist in the English language. The French language does not use the forward "r" sound, but instead uses the guttural "r." English speaking students of French know the difficulty of changing to an "r" that is made in the throat!

New muscle combinations are often more difficult for an adult to master. It is often more difficult for an adult to master a new language, especially a new accent, than a child, who has not yet formed muscular habits. Articulation exercises will help you master different dialects and different accents and make your English pronunciation more clear.

Muscles that are not flexible or strong will produce "lazy" consonants in daily conversation.

The first set of exercises will help you improve your articulation and also open up the point of release of your sound—your mouth. You can incorporate them into your daily routine of brushing your teeth. They take only a few minutes to complete and quickly produce remarkable results.

Like any exercise, frequency is the key. You should do the exercises at least three times a week, but you will experience results more quickly if you do them every day. Consistent practice will produce results!

LIP LICKING

OBJECTIVE: To stretch the tongue for ease of pronunciation.

EXERCISE:

- Lick your lips in large circles, reaching as far as possible in every direction.
- Reach for your nose, around to one ear, circle down and try to touch your chin.
- Work your way all the way around, like the hand of a clock.
- Circle one direction, 20 times.
- Reverse the direction and circle another 20 times.
- You will feel the workout!

THE FISH

OBJECTIVE: To stretch the lip muscles for the formation of m, b, and p.

EXERCISE:

This exercise is called "The Fish" because the exercise resembles the motion fish make with their mouths.

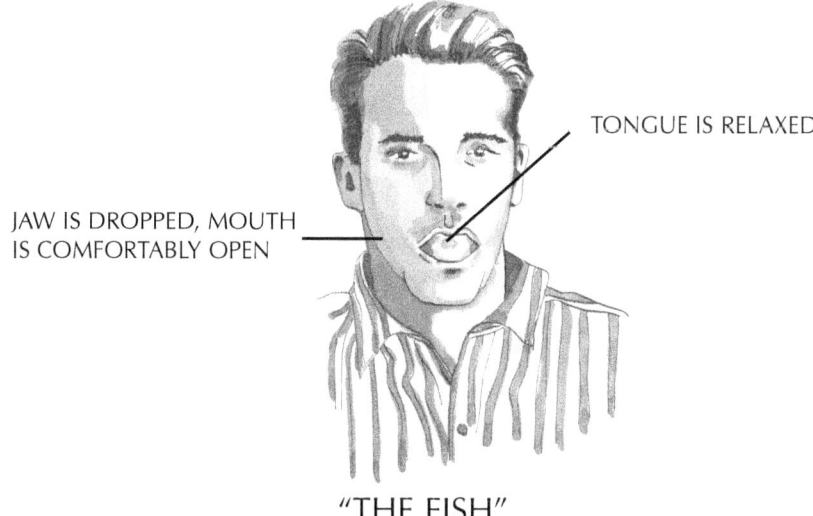

TONGUE IS RELAXED

JAW IS DROPPED, MOUTH IS COMFORTABLY OPEN

"THE FISH"

21

- Drop the jaw so the mouth is open by about two fingers in length.
- Maintaining this open position draw both lips together to form an "m."

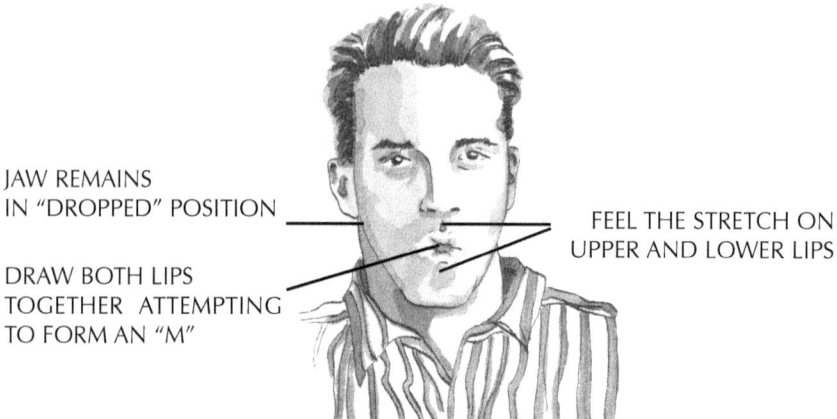

JAW REMAINS
IN "DROPPED" POSITION

FEEL THE STRETCH ON
UPPER AND LOWER LIPS

DRAW BOTH LIPS
TOGETHER ATTEMPTING
TO FORM AN "M"

- Feel the stretch on the upper and lower lips.
- Now repeat this. Relax your lips to an open position, and then bring them together to form a "m."
- It is important to keep your teeth apart in the original dropped jaw" position and let your lips do all the work.
- Repeat this 20 times each session.

EE-OO

OBJECTIVE: To stretch and strengthen the lip and cheek muscles for the clear formation of the sounds w, wh, ee, oo, ch and sh.

EXERCISE:

- Close the teeth as if "biting down" but without any pressure.
- Grin as broadly as you can, thinking of an "ee" sound.

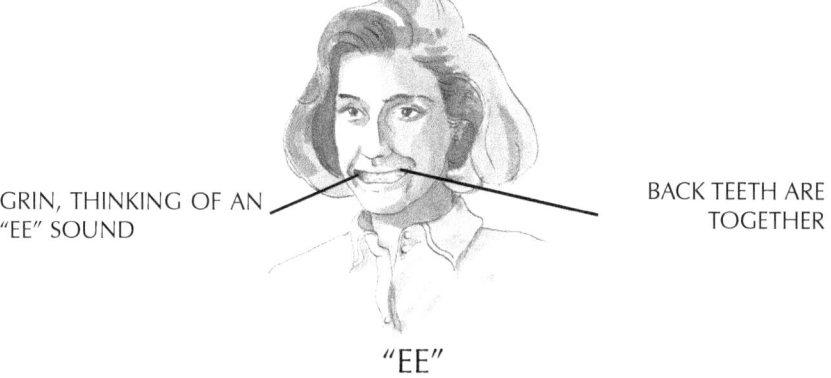

GRIN, THINKING OF AN "EE" SOUND

BACK TEETH ARE TOGETHER

"EE"

- Maintaining your "bite" position, pucker your lips thinking of an "oo" sound.
- This is not a voiced exercise. Just move your lips as if you were saying "ee" and "oo."
- Repeat this movement – ee, oo, ee, oo, - 20 times.
- Remember, it is important to keep the back teeth together and let the lips do all the work.

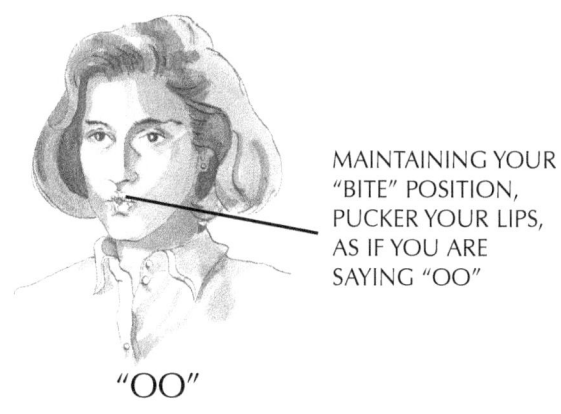

MAINTAINING YOUR "BITE" POSITION, PUCKER YOUR LIPS, AS IF YOU ARE SAYING "OO"

"OO"

TONGUE ROLLS

OBJECTIVE: To stretch the base of the tongue in order to release tension in the tongue root and throat. Tongue tension is the cause of the "necktie tenor", monotone delivery and prevents the release, or projection of sound.

EXERCISE:

- Drop the jaw in a relaxed position, as in "The Fish."
- Allow your tongue to relax on the floor of the mouth. It should look wide and flat.

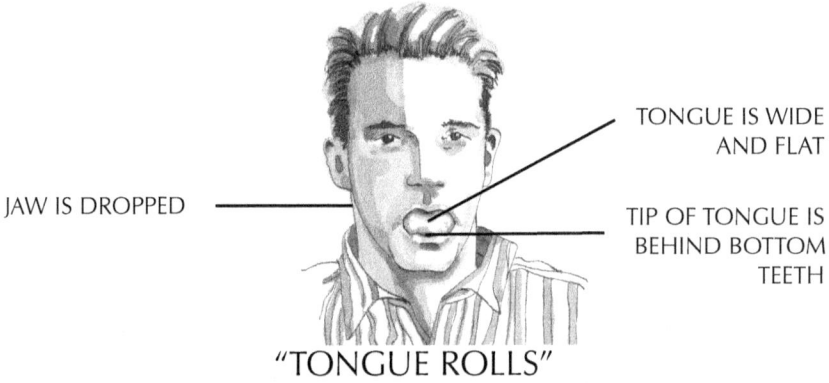

JAW IS DROPPED

TONGUE IS WIDE AND FLAT

TIP OF TONGUE IS BEHIND BOTTOM TEETH

"TONGUE ROLLS"

- Brace the tip of your tongue against the back of your bottom teeth and gently roll the middle of your tongue forward, out of your mouth.
- Maintaining a slightly open jaw position, repeat this out and in motion.

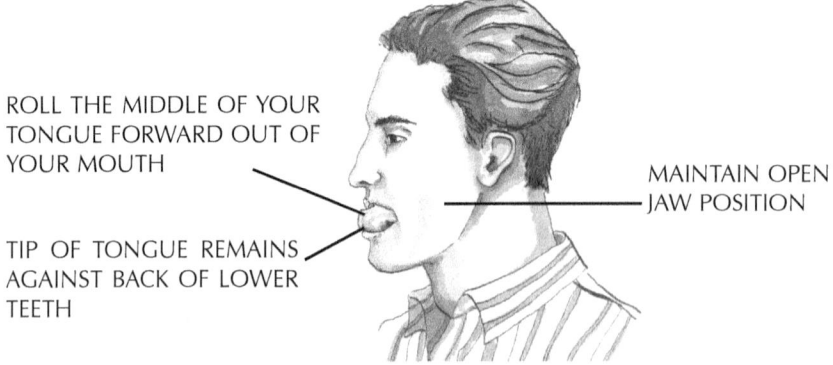

ROLL THE MIDDLE OF YOUR TONGUE FORWARD OUT OF YOUR MOUTH

TIP OF TONGUE REMAINS AGAINST BACK OF LOWER TEETH

MAINTAIN OPEN JAW POSITION

- Roll out, relax in, roll out, relax in, roll out, relax in...
- You will feel the stretch from the middle portion down to the root of your tongue.
- Do this slowly, 10 times.

"PEANUT BUTTER"

OBJECTIVE: To improve strengthen the tongue to improve clarity for the consonant sounds D, L, N, and T.

EXERCISE:
- Identify your "hard palate", the plate of bone which forms the roof of your mouth.
- Press your tongue on the ridge just on the inside of your upper teeth.
- Now, maintaining as much pressure as you can, slowly draw your tongue along the roof of your mouth from the front ridge to the back of your hard palate, as if you are trying to scrape off a thick layer of peanut butter.
- Then do this in reverse. Pressing your tongue against the roof of your mouth, draw your tongue from the back of your hard palate to the front ridge behind your front teeth.

THE YAWN

OBJECTIVE: This is something you have done many times in your life and is a terrific exercise for your voice. Yawning stretches and limbers your "soft palate", the soft domed area at the back of your throat where your uvula, or "punching bag" hangs. Yawning also opens up the size of the exit space for your voice that will allow your voice to be louder. This works on the same principle as a megaphone. The larger opening amplifies the sound.

The "yawn" is the basic position for later exercises on releasing sound and resonance, when you will be yawning out sound. Eventually you will have an open throat whenever you speak. It is helpful to use a mirror for this exercise until you identify what you are stretching and get used to the feeling of stretching it.

EXERCISE:

- Open your mouth and look toward the back of your throat, the way you would open your mouth and say "ah" for your doctor.
- Now yawn, watching the back of your throat.
- The area that forms a "dome" at the back of your throat will rise and you should feel a stretch in this area.
  This is your "soft palate."
- Practice lifting your soft palate with a yawn to identify what you have to do to lift and stretch this soft muscular area.
- Every time you yawn you are stretching the muscles that form this opening. The larger the opening at the back of your throat, the more your voice can be projected.
- Finally, when you yawn, keep your tongue forward and don't pull it back into your throat.

THE FLUTTER

OBJECTIVE: To relax the lips and cheeks for the formation of all consonants and enable more projection of sound.

EXERCISE:

- Take a breath and blow through your lips, making them flutter.
- Babies and horses do this.
- If you can't "flutter" your lips, take a bigger breath!
- If you still can't "flutter" you may be tensing your lips and cheeks to "blow."
- Don't "blow" the air out. Your lip muscles must be relaxed.
- If you still can't flutter your lips may be too tight at this time.
- The other exercises will help loosen up your lip and cheek muscles.
- Keep practicing your "flutter" at each session.

BREATHING

Breathing is an involuntary process. We breathe all the time without thinking about it. You might be tempted to skip this chapter. DON'T! Proper breathing is the key to phrasing, volume, and the overall quality of your voice. Your breath is the power source for your voice. This chapter is the foundation for the rest of the exercises, which target the other components of your voice. Your breath fuels your resonance, sound projection, and phrasing.

When the breathing muscles are weak, the muscles of the throat, jaw, lips, and tongue have to work harder to compensate for the lack of support. This results in a vocal tone that is thin and constricted. The breath must be free and supportive for the voice to reach its potential.

Breath support plays an essential role in the phrasing of sentences. In speaking or singing, we have to take a quick breath and the rate of exhalation has to sustain the length of a phrase or sentence. Lack of breath support causes the speaker to run out of breath before finishing the sentence. This results in choppy sentences or weak, inaudible endings of sentences. Firm breath support and an even rate of flow makes a speaker "eloquent."

First of all, let's take a look at the way you breathe. Put this book down and sit for a moment, simply observing your breath. Which areas of your body move when you take a breath? Your stomach? Your chest? Your waist or shoulders? Which takes longer, inhaling or exhaling?

If most of the movement is in your stomach and waist you are exhibiting good breathing habits. If your chest or shoulders rise when you inhale, chances are you are not using your diaphragm when you breathe. (We will locate and discuss the elusive diaphragm in a moment).

There are several reasons why so many people breathe into their chest, one of which is the all too common practice of holding in the stomach! Posture also plays an important part in breathing. Poor posture doesn't allow the breath space to reach its full capacity. Sitting or standing with an erect torso is essential to proper breath support and good vocal production.

The diaphragm is a large, sheet-like muscle that supports and projects your voice. Imagine the diaphragm as a trampoline. If the canvas of a trampoline were loose then it would be difficult to bounce very high. The bouncing surface, when sprung at just the right tension and flexibility, is able to propel someone high into the air.

Take another moment and sit with "good posture." To find the correct posture imagine you are wearing a crown on your head. Once you have that image or feeling, think of lifting the crown up to the ceiling. Now breathe into the pit of your stomach, imagining the trampoline at the very bottom. This time you have more awareness of you breath space and you may have breathed deeper. Your awareness of the extent of your breath space is the first step toward using more of this space and improving your voice.

The exercises in this chapter help you establish correct breathing habits. They may take more thought and practice than other exercises in the book. Be patient. Remember that you don't have to wait to finish the whole book to acquire a better voice. With every exercise, you improve some aspect of your voice. You will soon experience changes in your speech and gain confidence with your developing skills and the way you project yourself.

BREATHING INTO THE DIAPHRAGM

OBJECTIVE: This exercise will help you establish a correct breathing pattern. From now on, this is the first exercise to do in your vocal routine. You can even practice this before getting out of bed in the morning. You will need a book.

EXERCISE:

- Lie down with your back on the floor, knees bent, feet flat on the floor.
- Arrange your position so that the small of your back is flat against the floor and your head is level and comfortable. This position of "good posture" is easier to establish on the floor!
- The objective is to create a straight, direct route between your breath space and your mouth.
- Place the book on the soft part of your stomach.
- Now, breathe comfortably, at your own rate, keeping the small of your back flat against the floor.
- On each inhalation, the book should rise.
- On exhalation, the book should lower.
- This indicates that you are breathing deeply into your diaphragmatic area, not into your chest.
- If you find that on inhalation only your chest moves then experiment with how you could breathe into the area that makes the book gently rise.
- After approximately three minutes, stand up and breathe, maintaining your "correct" posture and the breathing placement pattern you established on the floor.

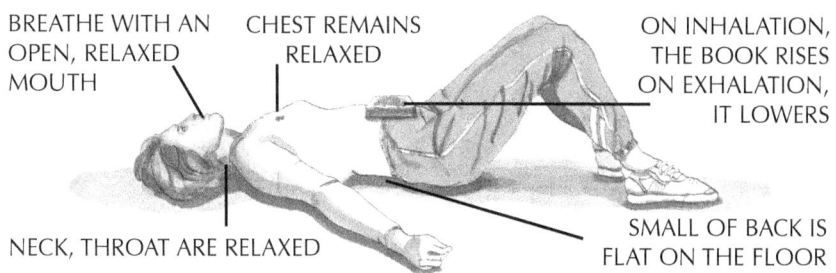

BREATHE WITH AN OPEN, RELAXED MOUTH

CHEST REMAINS RELAXED

ON INHALATION, THE BOOK RISES ON EXHALATION, IT LOWERS

NECK, THROAT ARE RELAXED

SMALL OF BACK IS FLAT ON THE FLOOR

"BREATHING INTO THE DIAPHRAGM"

THE SNAKE

OBJECTIVE: This exercise will increase the power of your breath exhalation and support. It is called "The Snake" because it involves a series of short, sharp hissing sounds.

EXERCISE:
- Sitting comfortably with "good posture", take a breath and "hiss" a short (one second) strong "hiss."
- Now "hiss" five times, on one breath.
- You should feel the muscles around your middle, back and seat working to expel this strong stream of air.
- Pace yourself with this one so you don't get dizzy!

LAUGHING

OBJECTIVE: Laughing is one of the best exercises for the diaphragm!

EXERCISE:
- Do it often!

EXPANDING
THE BREATHING
SOURCE

Most people only use a small portion of their total breathing capacity. The following exercises will increase your lung capacity when you breathe for more powerful projection power and more freedom in phrasing.

Before we start the exercises, sit on a dining chair or stool (not a soft armchair) and cough a few times. What do you feel when you cough? Where? Chances are you felt your waist, stomach, sides, and your seat muscles as well. You can feel the extent of the muscles involved in sending breath out of your body when your body contracts. The muscles all around the waist, stomach, and all the way down to the posterior are used involuntarily when you cough or sneeze! They will all play a part in your breathing exercises and eventually in the sounded exercises.

Because the muscles you use for breathing can't be "seen", it will be important to read and listen to the instructions, then visualize or feel what is happening inside your body. The exercises are described using images and the diagrams will also help you understand how to perform each exercise.

THE BALLOON

OBJECTIVE: "The Balloon" will expand your breath capacity.

EXERCISE

- Lie on the floor, as illustrated.
- Drop your jaw to an open mouth position, as in "The Fish."
- Inhale and imagine your breath entering a large balloon that is located down inside your body.
- This balloon is very elastic and expands in every direction.
- Imagine not just a party balloon, but also one of those big round punching bag balloons you may get at a summer fair.
- On inhalation, your breath will expand this balloon in all directions.
- The balloon expands:
- Down to your feet.
- Out the sides of your ribs.
- Down into the floor through your back.
- Up to the ceiling through the soft part of your stomach.
- Relax and exhale, letting your breath fall out of you all at once, allowing the balloon to collapse.
- Now, with the awareness that your breathing space can expand in all directions, make the balloon bigger with each inhaled breath.
- Remember, it expands in all directions.

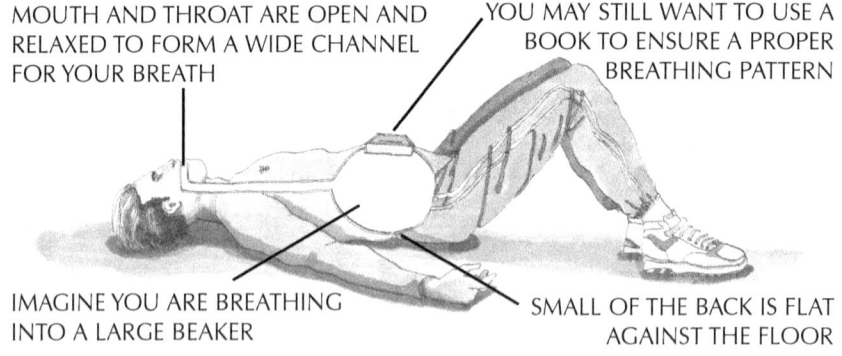

MOUTH AND THROAT ARE OPEN AND RELAXED TO FORM A WIDE CHANNEL FOR YOUR BREATH

YOU MAY STILL WANT TO USE A BOOK TO ENSURE A PROPER BREATHING PATTERN

IMAGINE YOU ARE BREATHING INTO A LARGE BEAKER

SMALL OF THE BACK IS FLAT AGAINST THE FLOOR

"THE BALLOON"

SIDE STRETCH

OBJECTIVE: To stretch the muscles along your ribs, further expanding your breath capacity.

EXERCISE:

- Stand with your feet a comfortable distance apart, knees slightly bent.
- Reach with your right hand over your head to your left side, while keeping your hips, shoulders, and head all in line.
- Use your left hand as a support on your thigh while maintaining this position.
- Now breathe deeply into the side that is being stretched, to a count of five.
- Direct your breath to the part of your rib cage that is being stretched.
- Think of a balloon on that side of your ribs, filling up with air.
- Breathe slowly into this side, five times.
- Return to an upright position and feel the difference between your right and left side when you breathe.
- Now repeat the process, stretching the left side.

The first chapters of this book have provided a foundation to help you gain the most benefit from the more advanced, sounded exercises in the following chapters. Again, I can't stress enough, the importance of breathing exercises in vocal development. Your breathing is your power source and it is important that you practice these exercises regularly to experience changes. Think of your breath often. Practice your deep breathing when riding the bus, watching television or sitting at the dinner table. The more you practice these exercises, the more quickly you will gain results!

BREATHING INTO THE BACK

OBJECTIVE: To increase the breath space in the lower back area.

EXERCISE:

- Sit on a dining room chair and lean over so that your chest meets your legs (or as close as you can manage). Then place your hands around your waist, at the back. Refer to the illustration.
- This position compresses the stomach area so the air you breathe has to displace the back muscles.
- Imagine a ballon that expands every time you inhale. Your hands will move as you take in a deep breath.
- Take five slow, deep breaths, feeling the stretch in your back muscles.
- If you have back problems or you don't find this position comfortable, take an intermediate position by resting your hands or elbows on your thighs for support.

STOMACH AREA IS CONSTRICTED, DISPLACING BREATH INTO THE BACK AREA

FEEL YOUR BACK AREA FILL WITH BREATH ON EACH INHALATION

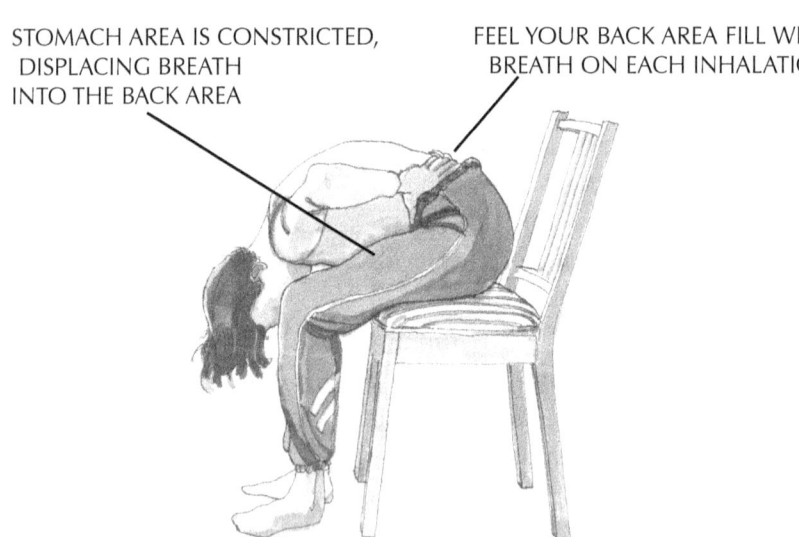

"BREATHING INTO THE BACK"

RELEASING
THE SOUND

So far, you have improved your power source, breath capacity, and limbered up the point of release—your mouth. Now you are going to put the two together and complete the whole vocal process by adding sound.

This chapter has three exercises that focus on releasing your voice through an open throat and eliminating tension or "holding" that prevents your voice from being projected to fill a room. These exercises will result in some reconditioning of the way you release your voice when you speak. Practicing this "release" of sound is a necessary step in preparation for the next chapter on resonance.

This is the first time you will be making sound. At the beginning, everyone feels a little self-conscious, as we are used to saying words, not making sounds. Find a place to be alone, where you won't be interrupted. With practice these exercises will become natural to you. These exercises are fundamental to the process of freeing your voice to become a clear, vibrant instrument.

SIGHING

OBJECTIVE: To form the habit of naturally releasing the voice through an open, unrestricted channel.

EXERCISE:

- Lie in "deep breathing" position.
- Relax and breathe in this position for about one minute, as you did with "The Balloon."
- Now, yawn a sigh of relief.
- Think of lying in a warm bathtub, on a beach, or somewhere else that triggers a response of relaxation and relief.
- At this point, you can review "The Yawn" if necessary.
- Next, you are going to add sound or tone to the yawn.
- Take a breath and release a voiced sigh, comfortably within your vocal range "aaaahhhh."
- You are essentially releasing a voiced sigh out of your body, through a flow of breath.
- All you have to do is relax and exhale an "aaahhh" the way you do when you "voice" a yawn when you are tired.
- When this happens your throat is open, your soft palate is raised, and your tongue and throat stretch to form a large opening.

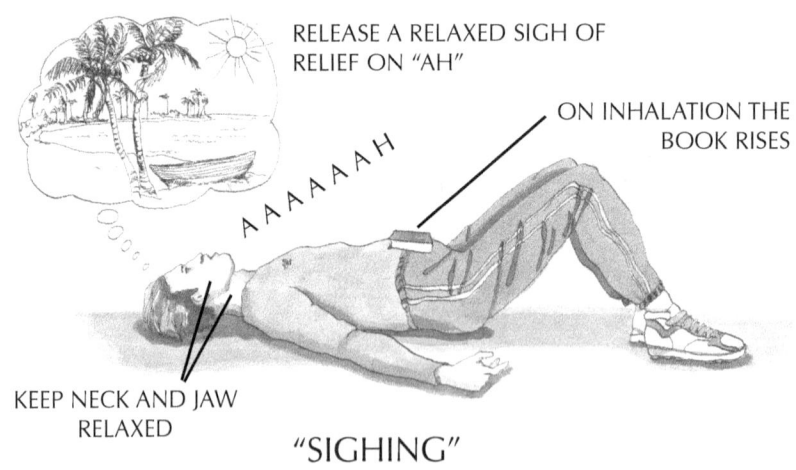

RELEASE A RELAXED SIGH OF RELIEF ON "AH"

ON INHALATION THE BOOK RISES

AAAAAAH

KEEP NECK AND JAW RELAXED

"SIGHING"

- Although it takes some explaining, don't make it out to be any more complicated than simply relaxing and releasing a sigh of relief.
- The following diagram illustrates the "aaahhh" in terms of sound.

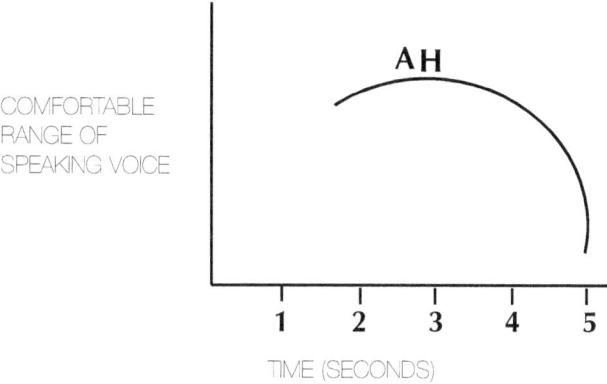

IMPORTANT NOTES:

1. It is important not to hold your breath before you start your "sigh". Breathe in, breathe out, and sound just happens to come out with the breath.
2. Do not use a "glottal attack" at the start of the sigh. A glottal attack, for example, is used at the beginning of the word "eye." The vocal cords close and hold back air. When the cords part, they vibrate as the air is released and tone is suddenly produced.
3. The sigh, or "aaaahhhh" in this exercise should be released the way you would say "high". At the beginning of this word, the vocal cords are open and remain open for the duration of the word.

CAR SOUNDS

OBJECTIVE: This exercise helps voice projection and develops more inflection or range of tone in your speaking voice.

EXERCISE:
- Flutter your lips by blowing through a "brrr" sound.
- Babies and horses do this.

- This time, do it with sound so you sound like a motor.
- Provide the "sound effects" for starting a car.
- Now send the car up the hill and down the hill.
- Do this fluttering up and down in pitch as long as you can.
- You will feel the workout!

You may find you can produce higher tones or "notes" while fluttering your lips than you can normally produce in speaking or singing. This is because your sound is being directed forward to the lips, nose, and sinus cavities and the muscular control in the throat is reduced or eliminated.

SHAKING OUT THE SOUND

OBJECTIVE: To release the voice in an uncontrolled manner in order to break the habit of "holding in" the voice. The exercise may seem awkward at first, as we are not used to "letting go." After "shaking out your sound" you will find your voice flows out of you. Your voice may also seem deeper and louder.

EXERCISE:
- In a standing position, feet shoulder width apart, raise your arms above your head.
- While sighing (refer to the "Sighing" exercise if necessary) let your shoulders and arms go limp like a rag doll.
- As your arms fall to your sides, bend each knee alternatively so your body gets a bouncing movement going from side to side.
- By bouncing from side to side you will be "shaking the sound out" of your body.
- There will be jerks in the sound as your musculature "lets go" of the control over the release of your voice.
- These jerks will sound like the jerks in your voice that would occur if you tried to talk during a bumpy car ride.
- If your sigh is smooth then you are not bouncing enough to let go of the sound and you are not gaining the benefits of the exercise.
- Practice five "shake-outs" in each session.

VOCAL RESONANCE

Vocal resonance determines the tone quality and the potential volume of your voice when you speak. A high degree of resonance is especially useful for anyone who speaks a lot, as resonance enables a voice to carry over a distance without strain. Volume can be achieved with less effort and so a resonant voice is less likely to get tired or go hoarse. You may have heard someone's voice deteriorate when they had to yell to be heard, or talk for a prolonged period of time.

The resonance of the human voice takes place in the cavities of the body. The chest cavities, mouth, nasal, and head cavities all provide chambers where the sound we produce can be amplified by "bouncing around" inside. The size and structure of your body cavities as well as the emotional responses of the muscles surrounding these cavities determine your voice. Tense muscles inhibit the vibration and resonance in the body cavities. Also, the way you direct the sound to these resonating chambers determines the degree of resonance in your voice; hence, your vocal characteristics.

Sometimes the sound is distributed unevenly in these resonating cavities and the voice becomes distorted. For example, a nasal voice is the result of directing too much sound into the nasal and sinus cavities and can be quite annoying to listen to. On the other hand, when the sinus and nasal cavities are blocked during a head cold the voice sounds distorted in a different way. Vibrations that are usually directed to the nose and sinus passages are being displaced to the mouth. Another example of voice placement is when we hear a voice of "authority." Our society's definition of an authoritative voice is one with well-developed chest resonance. You may recall the voices of newscasters, some professors and ministers, and certain actors who play roles of "authority."

Resonance gives your voice its appealing qualities and characteristics—it is essential to develop all your areas of resonance for a well-rounded, expressive voice that is interesting to listen to. The exercises in this chapter will help you develop a strong, well-balanced voice that is capable of expressing your personality, thoughts, and feelings.

Your main goals in developing resonance are:

1. To balance the distribution of sound in all your resonating spaces.
2. To increase your overall level of resonance.

If you think you need more of a certain quality in your voice then spend more time on the exercise that is designed to increase resonance in that particular area. For example, if you have a high or thin sound and you would like a voice with more depth or "authority", spend more time on the chest resonance exercise. If you already have a deep voice but need brighter tones to sound more exciting and less laid back, spend more time on the exercises for your upper resonating spaces.

PREPARATION NOTES FOR RESONANCE

In this chapter, reference is made to speaking "on tone" or changing "pitch." This refers to the frequency of the sound you are making, or in other words, making sounds that are high or low. We could call them "notes" except this is not quite appropriate as we are **speaking**, not singing. If you have any musical background you will understand what "higher" or "lower" tones refer to. However if these terms are new to you, the following explanation may help.

You use different tones in your voice all the time and your pitch changes according to the meaning of what you are saying. For example when asking a question, the pitch of the voice rises at the end of the sentence.

Where did he say he was going?

Or

How much does that cost?

The pitch rises at the end of each sentence. We automatically end the phrase on a higher tone to infer a question is being asked. Factual statements or orders tend to go down in pitch at the end of the sentence.

Tomorrow is going to be **hot.**

Or

Put that **down.**

Listen to the inflection in people's voices. Some people use many different tones in their speech and others speak close to monotone, or use only "one tone", with hardly any inflection at all. Practicing resonance exercises will make you more familiar with what your voice can do in order to go up and down in pitch and will develop your vocal range.

The exercises for breathing and releasing your sound will also help you acquire a voice with more inflection which will make your voice much more interesting to listen to. "CAR SOUNDS" is a particularly effective exercise to increase the range of inflection in your voice.

Always feel comfortable with the pitch you are using. If you voice a tone that causes tension in your throat, switch to a tone that is comfortable. In all the exercises, don't ever "push" the sound or attempt to be loud. Breathe in deeply, then release a free, relaxed sound. Relaxation is the key.

CONTENTED COW

OBJECTIVE: To encourage oral resonance and focus the voice to be "on tone". This exercise is especially good for the breathy voice or a voice that is soft-spoken. It also serves as a good warm-up for voices that tend to "crack" under pressure. Cows chew cud. In this exercise, you chew sound.

EXERCISE:
- Using a comfortable "tone" in your natural speaking range, say the word "home", closing your lips to form the "mmm" and sustain this "hum."
- While humming, chew this hum, keeping the lips closed.
- Think of "chewing the sound", keeping your lips together.
- Feel the vibrations move around in your mouth as you do this.
- Think of the sound made by a large bumblebee.
- Continue chewing the sound until you start to run out of breath. This is not a breathing exercise and you should not try to sustain the sound after your breath supply starts to run out.
- Repeat this chewing on different tones that are in the range of your speaking voice, ten times.

TARZAN

OBJECTIVE: To develop resonance in the chest cavities. Chest resonance gives the voice warmth and also lends an "authoritative" quality to speech. Many people try to push their voices down to sound deeper, which results in a false voice that sounds unnatural. After doing this exercise, record your voice mail and hear the difference!

EXERCISE:
- In a standing position, tilt your head back very slightly and drop your jaw.
- Take a breath and release a sustained "aaaahhhh" as you did in "SIGHING."
- Use all the principles from the sighing exercise, keeping an open channel from your breathing source to your mouth.

- Keep your mouth wide-open, jaw dropped.
- While sighing, pound your chest, "Tarzan style."
- Pound up and down your sternum or chest bone and across the top, from shoulder to shoulder.
- Pound hard enough to cause little "jerks" or "bumps" in your sound. The objective is to encourage vibrations, not bruise your chest!
- Say "aaaahhhh" again, this time on a slightly lower tone, and pound your chest again.
- You can also pound the lower part of your ribs at the side and back of your rib cage, if you can reach.
- If you can find someone to pound your back this will help encourage vibrations in the upper back part of your chest cavity as well.
- Repeat this sighing while pounding ten times.
- When you have finished this exercise, say something out loud and feel the difference in your voice.
- This exercise produces results quickly but don't overdo it!

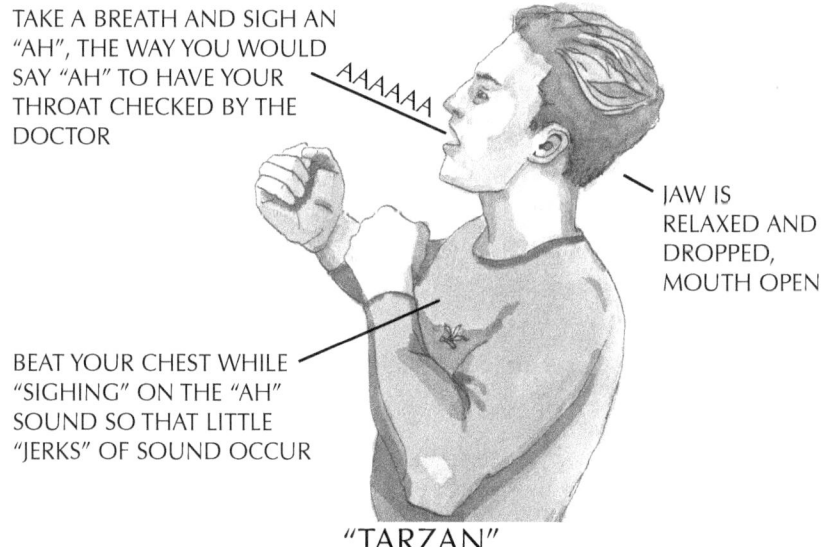

TAKE A BREATH AND SIGH AN "AH", THE WAY YOU WOULD SAY "AH" TO HAVE YOUR THROAT CHECKED BY THE DOCTOR

AAAAAA

JAW IS RELAXED AND DROPPED, MOUTH OPEN

BEAT YOUR CHEST WHILE "SIGHING" ON THE "AH" SOUND SO THAT LITTLE "JERKS" OF SOUND OCCUR

"TARZAN"

MEE-MEE

OBJECTIVE: To develop nasal resonance. Nasal resonance gives the voice brightness and helps the voice carry across a room with a sharp, crisp quality. This exercise adds excitement to dull voices.

EXERCISE:

- Sniff some air quickly, feeling the cool air pass through your nasal passages.
- Having mentally registered the places where the air rushed through, hum into this area.
- Feel the vibrations in the spaces where you felt the cool air.
- Practice this "humming into your nose" so that it is comfortable and automatic.
- Now turn the "mmm" into a "mee" with a smile.
- Think of the sound coming from the bridge of your nose.
- Crinkle your nose or place a finger on the bridge of your nose to help this happen.
- If you have trouble feeling the vibrations in your nose, sniff air through your nasal passages again to feel where you want the vibrations to occur.
- You could also flatten your tongue against the roof of your mouth to help channel the tones up into your nasal passages.
- Now say "meemeemeemeemeemeemee..." all run together on one exhalation, until you start to run out of air.
- Repeat the process on a slightly higher pitch.
- Do this ten times on tones that are comfortable for you.
- Remember, the whole time you are focusing the sound into your nose.
- When you have finished, speak out loud and listen to the changes in your voice.

THE MOSQUITO

OBJECTIVE: To encourage resonance in the sinuses and the skull.

EXERCISE:

- Get down on your hands and knees.
- Place your elbows on the ground and relax your head between your arms.
- This upside-down position helps the vibrations to drop into your head and sinus spaces as well as your nose.
- Take a big breath and hum.
- Think about the sound coming out of the top of your head.
- The hum will be small and high, like the sound of a mosquito.
- Raise your eyebrows and smile, keeping your lips closed while humming.
- This raises your soft palate and helps get the sound up into your head.
- It is important to let your head hang loosely.
- Do not hold your head up with your neck muscles.
- Hum on tones that are higher pitches in your voice.
- Repeat this five times, then stop, sit up and take a rest.
- Repeat five more hums, providing your voice doesn't feel tight or tired.
- We have to pace workouts on the higher pitches.

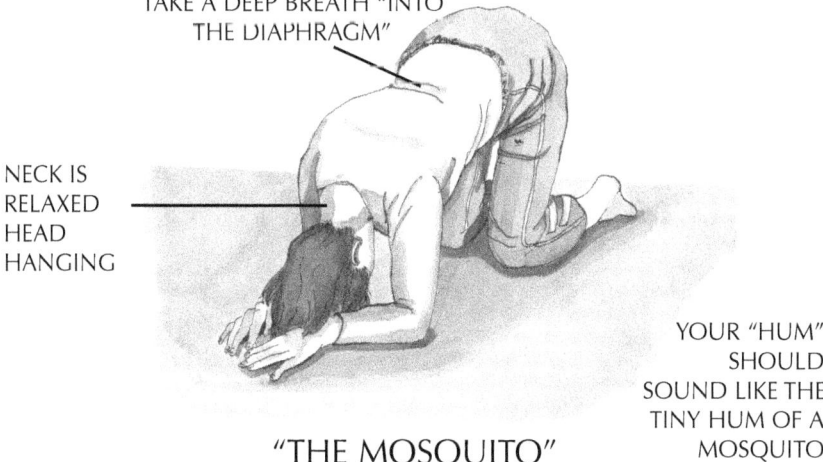

TAKE A DEEP BREATH "INTO THE DIAPHRAGM"

NECK IS RELAXED HEAD HANGING

YOUR "HUM" SHOULD SOUND LIKE THE TINY HUM OF A MOSQUITO

"THE MOSQUITO"

"And it is plain to me that eloquence, like swimming, is an art which all people might learn, though so few do."

Ralph Waldo Emerson

PHRASING ~ PUTTING IT ALL TOGETHER

Your breath control, tone quality, and variation of pitch will continue to improve as you work through the program. The rhythm and pacing of your voice is also essential to effective speaking. The following lists some common faults and how to remedy them.

1. Eliminate all non-verbal sounds like "em", "uh" and unnecessary words such as "like" and "you know". If you have to break to think for a moment, use a pause instead. Pauses make your speech more interesting. Trust that people will wait to hear what comes next!

The primary cause of "em" and "uh" is the way breath is used in the phrasing of sentences. Strong breath support will enable you to speak to the end of sentences without running out of air and filling in the break with "uh." CAR SOUNDS is an excellent exercise to achieve breath support in phrasing.

Also, reading aloud every day will help you develop the habit of speaking in full sentences. Choose a few paragraphs from the newspaper, a magazine, or other material you enjoy reading and read aloud. Take a breath before the sentence and speak in a long, fluid phrase until you come to the full stop or period. Take another full breath and speak right to the end of the sentence. Reading aloud is an excellent way to develop a fluid delivery.

2.   Don't have a "stage" voice. You should sound natural—like yourself. Take a breath, deliver your material and get your ideas across.

Trust the exercises to take care of the technical aspects of your voice. Your phrasing and tone quality will improve with the voice exercises in this book. When you speak, it is important to keep your focus on what you are saying, not what you sound like!

3.   It is a habit—of many speakers—to break up—their sentences —in odd places—through speech patterns—they have picked up—along the way—or—through lack of—breath control—or a steady—fluent—thought process.

Listeners get tired of listening very quickly as they are required to expend continuous mental effort to follow what is being said. Again, reading aloud is an extremely effective way to recondition habitual phrasing.

4.   Other speakers stress or "punch out" too many words to make their point! This is a style that is adopted, perhaps, to show conviction but actually turns the listener off! Would you engage in a conversation with someone who shouts every word at you?

Very often people punch out their words to make sure they are coming across and being heard. Developing more resonance allows appropriate emphasis as the speaker is assured they are being heard.

5.   Avoid slurring words together to form different ones, such as "willy lettuce" rather than "will he let us." Mumbling or slurring words can give a false impression of apathy or laziness.

The articulation set of exercises will ensure your consonants are crisp and clear.

You can also read aloud, over-enunciating the words until your mouth moves naturally to articulate the sounds.

PRE-SPEECH VOCAL WARM-UPS

When you encounter a really good speaker you may think they just walk out on stage, take the podium, microphone, or TV mark and talk. That's how natural it should appear, but it actually takes a lot of preparation to achieve that professional effect. In addition to rehearsing their dialogue or text, the good speaker has taken time to warm up, both physically and mentally.

The best professional speakers do warm-ups before they are required to address an audience. Warm-ups set your voice in good form so that your sound will be expressive, dynamic, and carry well. A full warm-up on the day you are to speak should include:

ARTICULATION

- THE FISH
- EE-OO
- TONGUE ROLLS
- LIP LICKING*
- THE YAWN*

BREATHING

- THE BALLOON
- SIDE STRETCH
- BREATHING INTO THE BACK*

RELEASING SOUND

- SIGHING
- CAR SOUNDS*
- SHAKING OUT THE SOUND

RESONANCE

- TARZAN*
- CONTENTED COW
- MEE-MEE*

* *Indicates the exercises to choose if you only have time to do a quick warm-up.*

By doing these pre-speech warm-up exercises, you will speak with the best vocal quality possible. The whole routine takes less than ten minutes. The "quick" version will take less than three minutes. Notice that the strengthening exercises have been omitted as they can cause muscular tension. On the day you are required to speak, you should concentrate on relaxing and releasing your voice. You can warm up at any time of the day when you are going to speak, but the closer you are to your actual "performance", the better.

As you get closer to the time you have to speak, nerves can affect your breathing pattern and cause tension in your body. This can affect your voice and your performance. The following exercises will help you to deal with these nerves.

DEEP BREATHING

In a sitting position, breathe deeply into your diaphragm and back on a slow count of three. Then, exhale completely. On each exhalation, consciously relax all the muscles in your body so you give more weight to the chair on each exhalation. You can practice this even while you are sitting and waiting to go and speak.

RELAXING THE NECK AND SHOULDERS

Shrug your shoulders, keeping them as high as they will go for a count of five, then circle them backwards and down, returning them to a resting position. Repeat this five times. Now lower your head forward so your chin reaches your chest and you feel a stretch at the back of your neck and upper back.

Slowly circle your head to the right until your ear is in line with your right shoulder, feeling the stretch on the left side of your neck. Then, slowly roll your head forward and around to the left until your left ear is in-line with your left shoulder. Roll to the center and back up. Don't forget to breathe while doing all this!

THE FACE

Lots of tension creeps into the face muscles so that by the time some people address an audience they have a frozen facial expression that doesn't come across as personable. Most people need to move their mouths more when they speak in a presentation. The articulation set of exercises is good to achieve this. Also, a yoga exercise called "The Lion" is excellent for relaxing the muscles in the face and brings some blood and energy into the face for more expression.

THE LION

While breathing in, scrunch your face as tightly as you can. Your eyes, mouth, cheeks, and nose should all be squeezed to the middle of your face. Then, while exhaling, open your eyes and mouth as wide as you can, sticking out your tongue at the same time. On an inhalation you scrunch up your face and on an exhalation you stretch and open your face up, sticking out your tongue. It looks crazy, but you can really feel the blood rush to your face. After five repetitions of "The Lion" you will look—and feel—much more relaxed.

PRESENCE

To address a large audience you need much more energy than you do when speaking to an individual or a few people in a room. You need a higher than usual personal energy level to reach your audience. "Energy" is an important trait that is taken for granted when present but sorely missed when absent. Energy plays a large role in that thing we call "presence."

Imagine the way you would walk into a room and say "hello" after a sedentary activity like sitting through a dull meeting or quietly reading a book. Now compare that with the way you would say "hello" after you had just finished a game of squash, or had been swimming. Physical activity generates energy. This energy pervades your body language, your mood, and your voice.

Your "hello" in each of the above scenarios may be spoken at the same volume, in the same manner, but one "hello" will be carried over by your personal energy and the other "hello" will not. Light exercise and stretching before speaking will raise your energy level—something that gets your blood flowing without tiring you out.

Exercise or movement of some kind also channels your nervous energy into physical energy. This energy will give you "presence" and help you "take the room" from the moment you arrive. Ten minutes of stretching, swinging your arms in large circles while breathing deeply and/or the vocal exercises in this book will prepare you to step out there and speak in a relaxed, dynamic manner—with an energy that gives you "presence!"

VOCAL POWER EXERCISE PROGRAM

To help you follow a program to develop and maintain your voice, you can use the following exercise charts or incorporate vocal exercises into your existing daily routines.

The charts list the exercises with check-off columns. Practice each of the exercises listed in each routine, starting with routine #1. There are six columns. If you practice three times a week, you will complete routine #1 in two weeks. If you choose to practice every day, you will complete each routine in one week. Always take one day off practicing per week. You can choose how often you would like to practice but remember that you are forming new habits so it is important to practice regularly.

You may choose to incorporate these exercises into your daily routines. You can practice deep breathing before getting out of bed in the morning. Put your pillow aside and start with breathing into the diaphragm. Then do "the balloon." The articulation exercises can be done at least once a day when you brush your teeth. You have a mirror handy and you can wash your face after "lip licking"!

You will have to put aside some time for those exercises that require special concentration and certain body positions. You will certainly want to do the sounded exercises when you are alone and free to make noise.

The only rule is that you do breathing exercises before you do any exercise requiring sound. This is because you should establish your support, or power source, before you start vocalizing.

Always remember that you are exercising and that rest is a very important part of an exercise program. Remember to take off at least one day per week. Be kind to your voice, and your instrument will serve you well for many years to come.

You have now learned the Vocal Power Voice Development Program; a system used in broadcast journalism departments across North America. Through exercises in articulation, breathing, resonance, and projection, you have the tools to develop a dynamic voice that connects with people. As you practice the exercises, you will experience more of your personality and feelings being expressed in your voice and you will be able to project in a room with ease.

Over time, your voice will reach a new level of expression and power that will contribute to your ability to motivate and persuade. I trust you have enjoyed working through this book. The results should give you a great deal of satisfaction, both personally and professionally.

CHRISTINA KAYA

EXERCISE PROGRAM CHARTS

ROUTINE #1

* Articulation, establishing good breathing habits.

EXERCISE	1	2	3	4	5	6	7	8	9	10	11	12
THE FISH												
EE-OO												
THE FLUTTER												
TONGUE ISOMETRICS												
TONGUE ROLLS												
LIP LICKING												
THE YAWN												
BREATHING INTO THE DIAPHRAGM												

ROUTINE #2

* Continue articulation, breathing, add expanding the breath capacity.

EXERCISE	1	2	3	4	5	6	7	8	9	10	11	12
THE FISH												
EE-OO												
THE FLUTTER												
LIP LICKING												
THE YAWN												
BREATHING INTO THE DIAPHRAGM												
DIAPHRAGM WORKOUT												
THE BALLOON												
THE BALLOON SIDE STRETCH												
BREATHING INTO THE BACK												

ROUTINE #3

* Maintenance of articulation, breathing, and releasing sound.

EXERCISE	1	2	3	4	5	6	7	8	9	10	11	12
BREATHING INTO THE DIAPHRAGM												
DIAPHRAGM WORKOUT												
THE FLUTTER												
TONGUE ROLLS												
THE YAWN												
THE BALLOON												
SIDE STRETCH												
BREATHING INTO THE BACK												
SIGHING												
CAR SOUNDS												

ROUTINE #4

* Maintenance of articulation, breathing, releasing sound, increasing breath capacity.

EXERCISE	1	2	3	4	5	6	7	8	9	10	11	12
BREATHING INTO THE DIAPHRAGM												
THE BALLOON												
THE SNAKE												
TONGUE ROLLS												
SIGHING												
CAR SOUNDS												
TARZAN												
CONTENTED COW												
MEE-MEE												
TONGUE ISOMETRICS												
THE YAWN												
READ ALOUD (1 PAGE OF TEXT)												

ROUTINE #5

* Maintenance of articulation, breathing, and resonance.

EXERCISE	1	2	3	4	5	6	7	8	9	10	11	12
THE FISH												
EE-OO												
THE FLUTTER												
TONGUE ROLLS												
BREATHING INTO THE DIAPHRAGM												
DIAPHRAGM WORKOUT												
THE SNAKE												
THE BALLOON												
CAR SOUNDS												
CONTENTED COW												
TARZAN												
THE MOSQUITO												
READ ALOUD (1 PAGE OF TEXT)												

ROUTINE #6

* Balanced maintenance of breathing, resonance, and releasing sound.

EXERCISE	1	2	3	4	5	6	7	8	9	10	11	12
BREATHING INTO THE DIAPHRAGM												
THE BALLOON												
SIDE STRETCH												
THE SNAKE												
SIGHING												
CAR SOUNDS												
SHAKING OUT THE SOUND												
TARZAN												
CONTENTED COW												
MEE-MEE												
THE MOSQUITO												
READ ALOUD (1 PAGE OF TEXT)												

ROUTINE #7

MASTER LIST – FULL WORKOUT

EXERCISE	PAGE
LIP LICKING	21
THE FISH	21
EE-OO	23
TONGUE ROLLS	24
PEANUT BUTTER	25
THE YAWN	25
THE FLUTTER	26
BREATHING INTO THE DIAPHRAGM	29
THE SNAKE	30
LAUGHING	30
THE BALLOON	32
SIDE STRETCH	33
BREATHING INTO THE BACK	34
SIGHING	36
CAR SOUNDS	37
SHAKING OUT THE SOUND	38
CONTENTED COW	44
TARZAN	44
MEE-MEE	46
THE MOSQUITO	46
THE LION	55

Visit www.KayacoSeminars.com for seminar dates and locations:

The Blueprint for Business Presentation Design

Be the architect of your own design. Learn to use a proven system to quickly and consistently construct a clear, concise presentation that leads people to take action.

(One day.)

Presenting With Precision

Your guarantee of a polished, professional presentation with expert, customized coaching and exercises for your voice, gestures, eye contact and blocking (where to stand, when to move).

(One day. Prerequisite, "The Blueprint".)

The Science Behind Persuasion

Tangible techniques of persuasion using principles of hypnosis to incorporate influence into your daily personal and professional life.

(One day.)

From Fear to Confidence & Control

Conquer your fear of presenting and gain the feeling of confidence. Specifically for people who are required to speak in front of groups.

(One day.)

Other publications for your interest:

The Ink Drop Effect

Connecting Minds through Excellence in Communication

A concise resource to better understand the role expectations, timing and framing information has on achieving results.

Magicalinguistics

Secrets of Influence Using Hypnotic Language

Once upon a time, magical words or "incantations" were spoken aloud to cast spells. Words can seem like "spells" when they influence the thoughts, decisions and behaviour of others.

Visit www.KayacoSeminars.com

Watch for weekly episodes of:

1-Minute Magic Moments

and

12-minute Lunch'n Learns

www.ingramcontent.com/pod-product-compliance
Lightning Source LLC
Chambersburg PA
CBHW071245280526
45788CB00004B/1594